Cancer Metabolic Healing

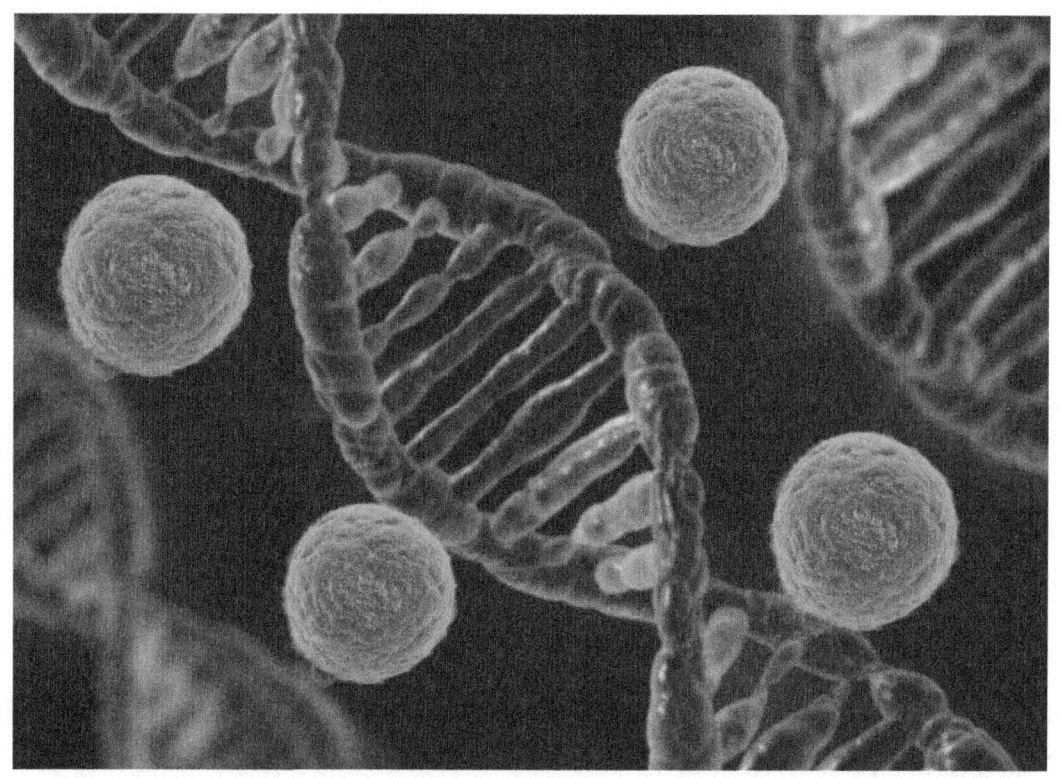

An Oncologist Revealing Metabolic And Nutritional Healing For Cancer Using Ketogenic Therapy (A Cancer Survivors' Guide)

Caroline Johnson

5-6

Introduction

7-9

Chapter 1: Introduction to the metabolic approach to treating cancer: exploring the link between cellular metabolism and cancer development

10-12

Chapter 2: Understanding the Warburg effect: a key characteristic of cancer cells and its implications for metabolic interventions

13-15

Chapter 3: Targeting cancer metabolism with lifestyle modifications: diet, exercise, and stress management as potential strategies for preventing and treating cancer

16-19

Chapter 4: Nutraceuticals as metabolic therapeutics for cancer: exploring the potential use of specific nutrients and food compounds in inhibiting cancer growth

20-22

Chapter 5: The role of fasting and calorie restriction in cancer treatment: examining the effects of reducing calorie intake on cancer cell metabolism and tumor growth

23-25

Chapter 6: Metabolic therapies for cancer: an in-depth look at treatments such as hyperthermia, photodynamic therapy, and hyperbaric oxygen therapy and their impact on cancer metabolism

26-28

Chapter 7: The microbiome and cancer: the influence of gut bacteria on metabolism and potential for targeted treatments

29-30

Chapter 8: Mitochondrial dysfunction in cancer cells: understanding the role of dysfunctional mitochondria in cancer development and exploring potential therapies targeting these organelles

31-33

Chapter 9: Integrative approaches to cancer treatment: the combination of conventional cancer treatments with metabolic interventions for a holistic approach to healing

34-38

Chapter 10: Clinical trials and future directions: reviewing current research on the metabolic approach to cancer treatment and potential directions for future studies.

39

Conclusion

Copyright © 2023 by Caroline Johnson

All rights reserved. No part of this publication may be reproduced, distributed, or transmitted in any form or by any means, including photocopying, recording, or other electronic or mechanical methods, without the prior written permission of the publisher, except in the case of brief quotations embodied in critical reviews and certain other noncommercial uses permitted by copyright law.

Introduction

Emily was an ambitious 28-year-old woman with a promising career as a lawyer. She had just gotten married to her college sweetheart and everything seemed to be falling into place. However, her world was turned upside down when she was diagnosed with breast cancer.

At the time of her diagnosis, Emily was devastated and scared. She knew that cancer was a serious disease and the treatment process was long and grueling. Her doctors recommended the standard treatment of chemotherapy, radiation, and surgery. Emily was determined to fight this disease with all her might, but she was also worried about the side effects of these treatments.

As she began her treatment, Emily experienced the debilitating side effects of chemotherapy. She felt nauseous, lost her appetite, and had no energy to do anything. Her hair started falling out and she could see the toll it was taking on her body. She started to question if she could continue with this treatment. That was when she stumbled upon a new approach to treating cancer – the metabolic approach.

Through research, Emily learned that cancer cells have a different metabolism compared to healthy cells. Cancer cells thrive on sugar and can't survive in an environment with limited sugar. The metabolic approach focuses on limiting the amount of sugar in the body through diet and other lifestyle changes, creating an environment that is not conducive for cancer cells to grow.

Excited and motivated, Emily immediately switched to a low-sugar and high-fat diet. She also incorporated exercise and stress-reduction techniques into her daily routine. In just a few weeks, she started to feel more energetic and her appetite returned. Her doctors were surprised at her improvements and suggested continuing with the standard treatment, but Emily was determined to stick with the metabolic approach.

Months went by and Emily's health continued to improve. Her tumor began to shrink and her energy levels were higher than ever before. After a year of following the metabolic approach, Emily's doctors were amazed to see that her cancer was completely gone. They couldn't believe it, and Emily was overjoyed. She had beaten cancer using a holistic and natural approach.

Emily's journey didn't end there. She became an advocate for the metabolic approach and started a support group for cancer patients looking for alternative treatments. She also went on to become a certified nutritionist, helping others with their journey to better health.

Looking back, Emily realized that cancer was a blessing in disguise. It allowed her to discover a new passion and a new way of life. She was grateful for the support of her family and friends, and for having the courage to follow her own path to recovery. Emily's experience showed her that there is no one-size-fits-all approach to treating cancer and that taking control of her own health was one of the best decisions she ever made…

Having cancer is not a death sentence, it can be treated with gradual process. Metabolic approach is one of the best ways to face cancer. This approach is not a difficult one. There are things you just need to adjust in your daily life. This book contains action steps for metabolic approach to cancer and all you need to do to gradually get rid of cancer completely. You too can fight this battle. I have had patients who has strive and conquered this cancer battle and you can fight it too with metabolic approach.

Chapter 1: Introduction to the metabolic approach to treating cancer: exploring the link between cellular metabolism and cancer development

Despite significant advancements in medical treatments, cancer remains one of the leading causes of death globally. Traditionally, cancer has been treated with surgery, chemotherapy, and radiation therapy. These treatments aim to destroy cancer cells or prevent them from growing and spreading. However, these treatments often have severe side effects, and cancer cells can develop resistance to them.

In recent years, there has been growing interest in a metabolic approach to treating cancer that aims to target the abnormal metabolism of cancer cells. The metabolic approach to treating cancer is based on the understanding that cancer cells have a distinct metabolism compared to healthy cells. This approach focuses on exploring the links between cellular metabolism and cancer development. Metabolism is the process by which cells convert nutrients into energy, and it is essential for the normal functioning and growth of cells. However, in cancer cells, this process is altered, leading to abnormal growth and division.

One of the key characteristics of cancer cells is their ability to proliferate rapidly and grow uncontrollably. This is due to a metabolic reprogramming that allows cancer cells to produce energy and building blocks for the cell's growth and division. This process is known as the Warburg effect, named after the scientist Otto War burg, who first described it in the 1920s. The Warburg effect is characterized by the increased utilization of glucose and production of lactic acid, even in the presence of oxygen. In healthy cells, energy production primarily occurs through the efficient breakdown of glucose in the presence of oxygen, known as aerobic respiration.

However, cancer cells rely on anaerobic respiration, or the breakdown of glucose without oxygen, to meet their energy demands. The Warburg effect also leads to the accumulation of metabolic byproducts, such as lactate and H^+ ions, in the tumor microenvironment. This creates an acidic and hypoxic environment, which promotes the growth and survival of cancer cells and is detrimental to healthy cells.

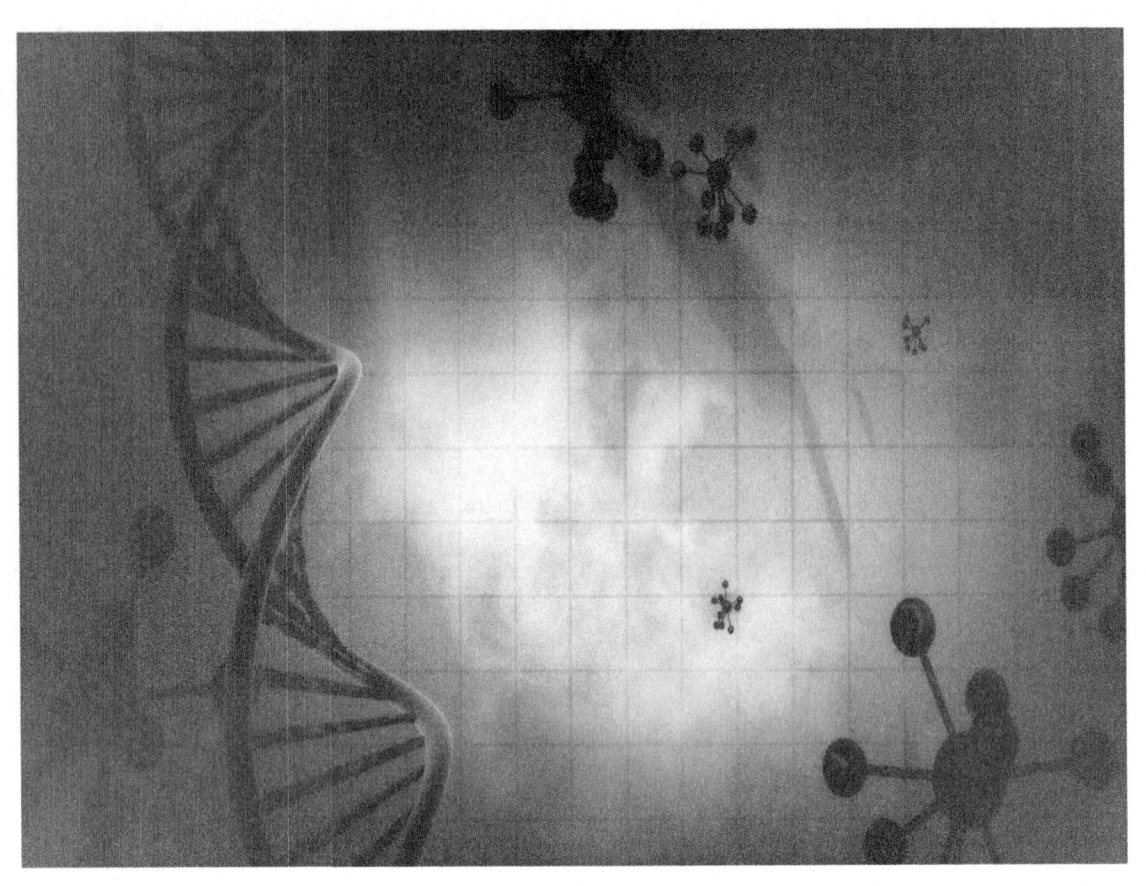

Additionally, this altered metabolism provides cancer cells with a growth advantage, as they can produce energy and building blocks more efficiently, allowing them to outcompete healthy cells. The metabolic approach to treating cancer aims to exploit these metabolic differences between cancer cells and healthy cells, with the goal of selectively targeting cancer cells while sparing healthy cells. One well-studied example of this approach is the use of the glucose analogue 2-deoxyglucose (2-DG) as a metabolic inhibitor. 2-DG blocks glucose uptake and inhibits glycolysis, the process by which glucose is converted into energy in cancer cells. As a result, cancer cells are deprived of the energy they need to grow and divide.

Various studies have shown promising results in using 2-DG in combination with other cancer treatments, such as chemotherapy and radiotherapy, to enhance their effectiveness and reduce side effects. In addition to targeting the Warburg effect, other metabolic pathways have also been identified as potential targets for cancer treatment. For example, researchers have found that some types of cancer cells are dependent on the amino acid glutamine for their growth and survival. Blocking glutamine metabolism has been shown to be effective in inhibiting cancer cell growth both in vitro and in animal studies.

Another emerging strategy in the metabolic approach to treating cancer is through the use of dietary interventions. It has been observed that dietary interventions, such as calorie restriction and fasting, can alter the metabolism of cancer cells and make them more sensitive to conventional cancer treatments. This is achieved by reducing the availability of glucose and other nutrients, which are necessary for cancer cell survival, while simultaneously promoting conditions that are detrimental to cancer cell growth. Studies have shown that incorporating these dietary interventions in combination with standard cancer treatments can improve treatment outcomes and reduce side effects.

Despite the promising evidence, the metabolic approach to treating cancer is still in its early stages and requires further research and clinical trials. One of the challenges in this approach is finding ways to selectively target cancer cells without harming healthy cells, as many metabolic pathways are also essential for normal cellular function.

Chapter 2: Understanding the Warburg effect: a key characteristic of cancer cells and its implications for metabolic interventions

The Warburg effect, also known as aerobic glycolysis, is a metabolic phenomenon whereby cancer cells preferentially utilize glycolysis for energy production, instead of the more efficient oxidative phosphorylation that takes place in normal cells. This increased reliance on glycolysis leads to a high rate of glucose consumption and lactate production, even in the presence of oxygen. This was first observed by the German physiologist Otto Warburg in the 1920s and has since become recognized as a key characteristic of cancer cells.

The Warburg effect represents a shift in the metabolism of cancer cells, as they rewire their energy production in order to support their rapid growth and proliferation. Unlike normal cells that rely on a mix of glycolysis and oxidative phosphorylation to generate energy, cancer cells predominantly use glycolysis even in the presence of oxygen. This process is less efficient than oxidative phosphorylation, but it allows cancer cells to rapidly produce ATP (the primary source of energy for cells) to support their high energy demand.

One of the main implications of the Warburg effect is that cancer cells require a constant supply of glucose in order to sustain their high rate of proliferation. This is why cancer cells take up glucose from the blood at a much higher rate than normal cells, making 18F-FDG positron emission tomography (PET) scans a useful diagnostic tool for detecting cancer.

Furthermore, the Warburg effect leads to the accumulation of lactate, a byproduct of glycolysis, in the tumor microenvironment. This creates an acidic environment that helps cancer cells evade immune detection and promotes their aggressive growth. Another important aspect of the Warburg effect is that it allows cancer cells to bypass normal regulatory processes that control cell growth. In normal cells, a process called oxidative phosphorylation regulates cell growth by controlling the availability of ATP.

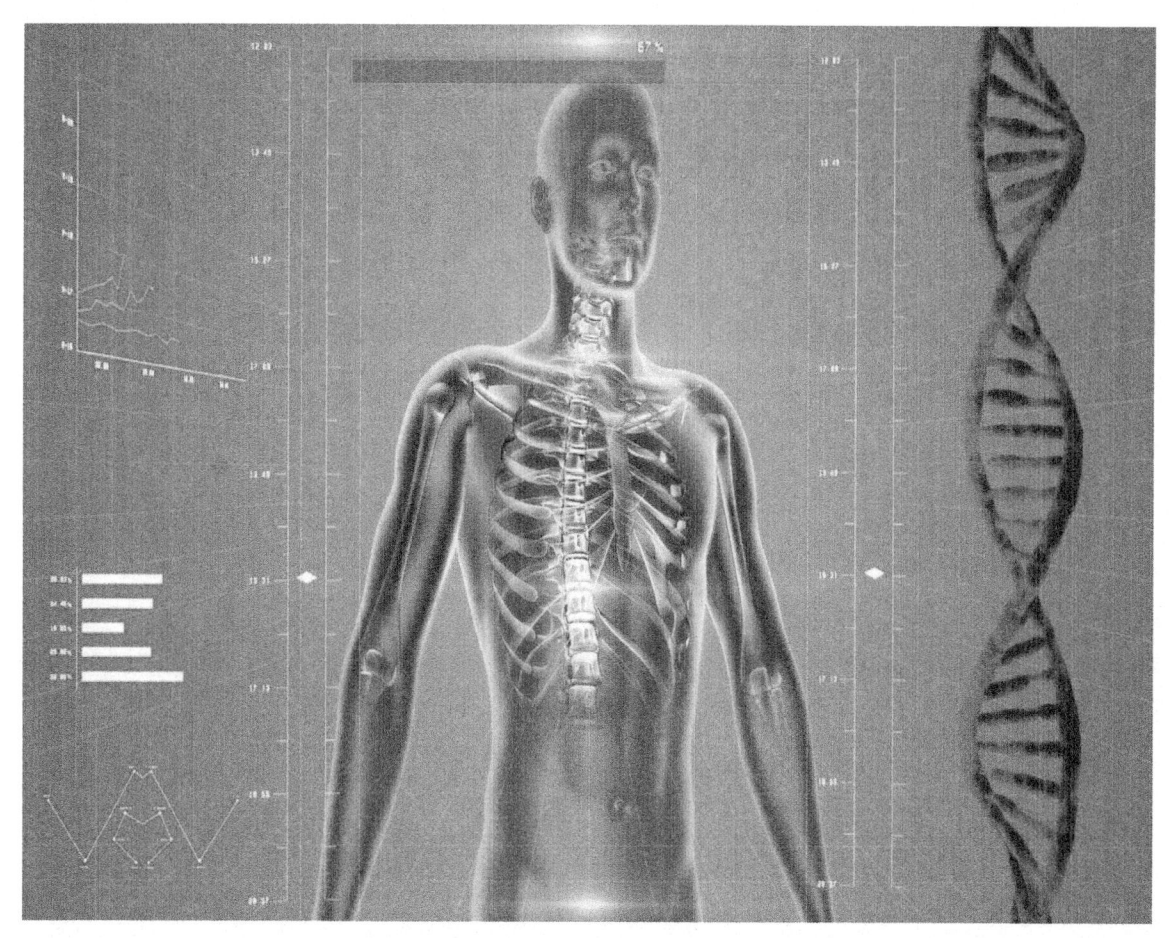

However, cancer cells that rely on glycolysis for energy production are able to bypass this process, leading to uncontrolled growth. The Warburg effect has also been linked to the development of resistance to chemotherapy and radiation therapy. Cancer cells that rely on glycolysis are less sensitive to these treatments, as they do not rely on oxidative phosphorylation for energy production. This creates a challenge in cancer treatment and highlights the need for targeted therapeutic approaches that can specifically target metabolic pathways in cancer cells.

Understanding the Warburg effect has also opened up new avenues for developing metabolic interventions as potential treatments for cancer. Researchers have identified various enzymes and pathways involved in the Warburg effect that can be targeted with drugs. For example, inhibiting the glycolytic enzyme, pyruvate kinase M2 (PKM2), has been shown to slow the growth of cancer cells and sensitize them to chemotherapy. Other interventions, such as targeting lactate transporters, have also shown promising results in inhibiting cancer cell growth.

The Warburg effect is a key characteristic of cancer cells and has significant implications for cancer diagnosis and treatment. Its role in promoting rapid energy production and cell growth has made it a major focus of research in the field of cancer biology. Understanding the mechanisms behind the Warburg effect opens up new opportunities for developing more effective and targeted therapies for cancer. Further research in this field may potentially lead to breakthrough treatments and improved outcomes for cancer patients.

Chapter 3: Targeting cancer metabolism with lifestyle modifications: diet, exercise, and stress management as potential strategies for preventing and treating cancer.

Cancer is a complex disease that involves abnormal growth and proliferation of cells in the body. While there are various factors that can contribute to the development of cancer, recent studies have shown that there is a strong connection between cancer and metabolism. This has led to the development of a new approach known as "metabolic therapy," which focuses on targeting cancer's metabolism in order to prevent and treat the disease. Lifestyle modifications, such as diet, exercise, and stress management, are some of the strategies that can be incorporated into metabolic therapy for cancer prevention and treatment.

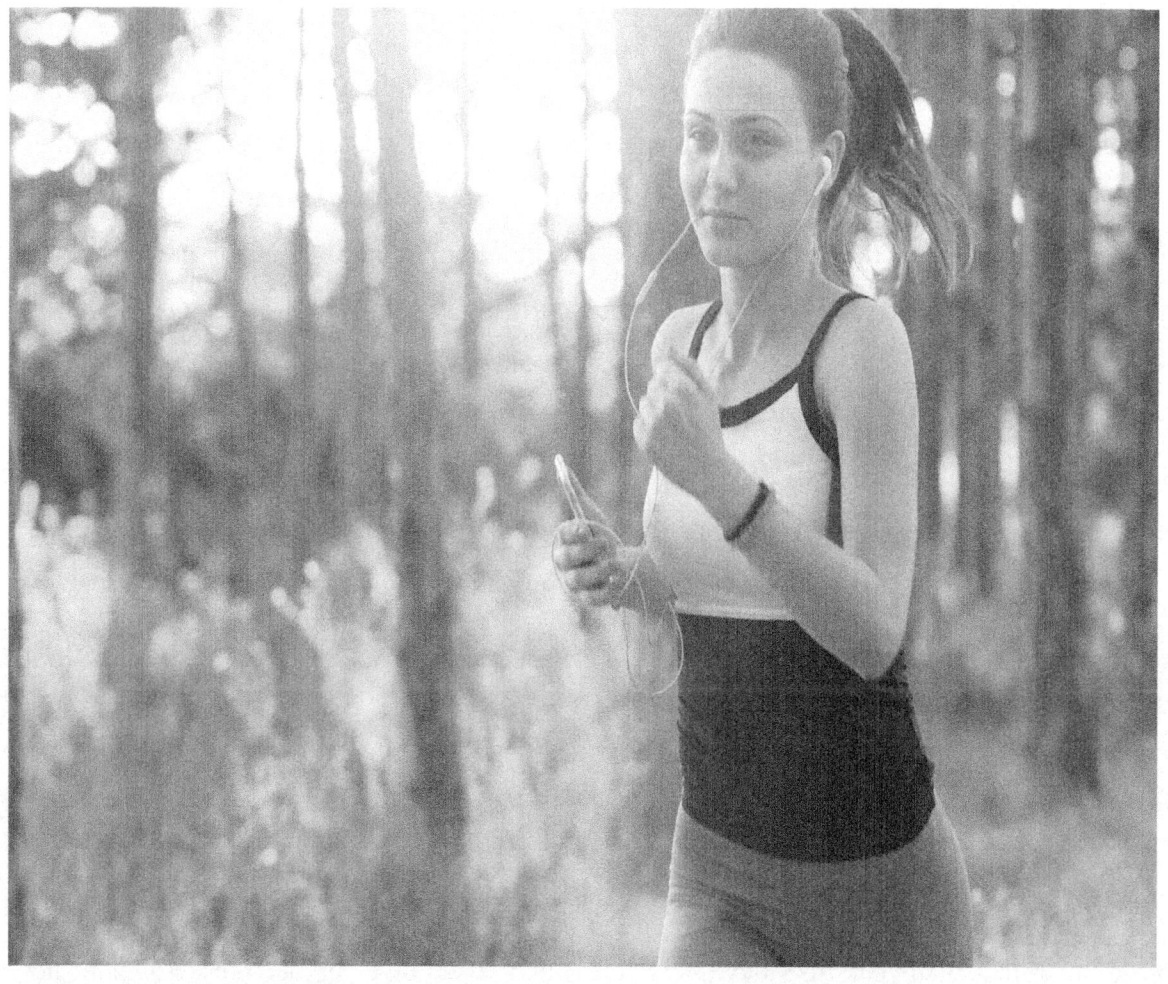

Diet plays a crucial role in our overall health, and it is no different when it comes to cancer. Studies have shown that certain dietary patterns can increase or decrease the risk of cancer. For instance, a diet high in processed and red meats has been linked to an increased risk of colorectal cancer, while a diet rich in fruits, vegetables, and whole grains has been associated with a lower risk of developing various types of cancer. Therefore, adopting a healthy and balanced diet can be a powerful tool in preventing cancer.

One dietary approach that has gained popularity in cancer prevention and treatment is the ketogenic diet. This diet has to do with consuming good amounts of healthy fats, considerable amounts of protein, and low amounts of carbohydrates. The ketogenic diet forces the body to use fat as its primary source of energy instead of glucose. Cancer cells, on the other hand, rely heavily on glucose for their energy needs, and by limiting their access to glucose, the growth and proliferation of cancer cells can be inhibited. Additionally, research has shown that the ketogenic diet can help reduce inflammation in the body, which is a major contributing factor in the development and progression of cancer.

In addition to diet, exercise has also been shown to have a role in cancer prevention and treatment. Regular physical activity is known to boost the immune system, improve cardiovascular health, and regulate hormone levels, all of which can help prevent and fight cancer. Additionally, exercise can help maintain a healthy weight, which is crucial as obesity has been linked to an increased risk of various types of cancer.

Stress and cancer have a bidirectional relationship, where stress can contribute to the development of cancer, and cancer itself can cause significant emotional distress. It is important to manage stress levels to support overall health and well-being, and this is especially important for cancer patients. When the body is under stress, it produces higher levels of cortisol, a hormone that can promote tumor growth and spread. Additionally, managing stress through practices such as mindfulness meditation, yoga, and breathing exercises can help improve emotional well-being and support the immune system.

Incorporating lifestyle modifications like a healthy diet, exercise, and stress management into cancer treatment plans can also have significant benefits. For example, the ketogenic diet has been shown to enhance the effectiveness of chemotherapy and radiation therapy while protecting healthy cells from damage. Regular exercise can also improve treatment outcomes by reducing fatigue and improving quality of life. And stress management techniques can help cancer patients cope with the emotional impact of the disease and its treatment.

Targeting cancer metabolism with lifestyle modifications is a promising approach for preventing and treating cancer. A healthy diet, regular exercise, and stress management can not only reduce the risk of cancer but also support traditional cancer treatments. It is important to consult with a healthcare professional, registered dietitian, or certified fitness trainer to create an individualized plan that works best for each person. By incorporating these lifestyle modifications into daily routines, individuals can take an active role in their cancer prevention and treatment journey and improve their overall health and well-being.

Read More Books By Caroline Johnson
You can fight cancer
How to Starve breast cancer
Recipes for Delicious Christmas meals
Grow your mind
Teenage Sexuality

Chapter 4: Nutraceuticals as metabolic therapeutics for cancer: exploring the potential use of specific nutrients and food compounds in inhibiting cancer growth

Cancer is a complex disease that arises from the uncontrolled growth of abnormal cells in the body. It is the second leading cause of death worldwide and current treatments often have significant side effects and limited success in preventing or curing the disease. As a result, researchers are constantly seeking new approaches to combat cancer, including the use of specialized nutrients and food compounds as metabolic therapeutics. These compounds, known as nutraceuticals, have shown promising potential in inhibiting cancer growth and may serve as a valuable addition to traditional cancer treatments.

Nutraceuticals are naturally occurring compounds found in food that have medicinal properties. They are able to interact with metabolic pathways in the body and have been shown to have an impact on cancer cell growth and proliferation, as well as the development of cancer cells at the molecular level. Some of the most widely studied nutraceuticals for cancer prevention and treatment include polyphenols, carotenoids, fatty acids, and phytochemicals.

Polyphenols, which are found in a variety of foods including fruits, vegetables, and spices, have been extensively studied for their anti-cancer properties. These compounds have been shown to inhibit the growth of cancer cells, induce cell death, and prevent the formation of new blood vessels that supply tumors with nutrients and oxygen. For example, curcumin, a polyphenol found in turmeric, has been found to have potent anti-cancer effects in various types of cancer, including colon, breast, and prostate.

Carotenoids, which are pigments responsible for the red, orange, and yellow colors in plants, have also been studied for their potential role in cancer treatment and prevention. They act as antioxidants and have been shown to inhibit the growth of cancer cells, induce cell death, and prevent DNA damage that can lead to cancer development. Some carotenoids, such as lycopene found in tomatoes, have also been found to have a protective effect against specific types of cancer, such as prostate cancer.

Fatty acids, particularly omega-3 fatty acids, have been extensively studied for their role in cancer prevention and treatment. These healthy fats are found in foods such as fish, nuts, and flaxseed, and have been shown to have anti-inflammatory and anti-cancer effects. Studies have demonstrated that omega-3 fatty acids can inhibit cancer cell growth, induce cell death, and enhance the effects of chemotherapy and radiotherapy treatments.

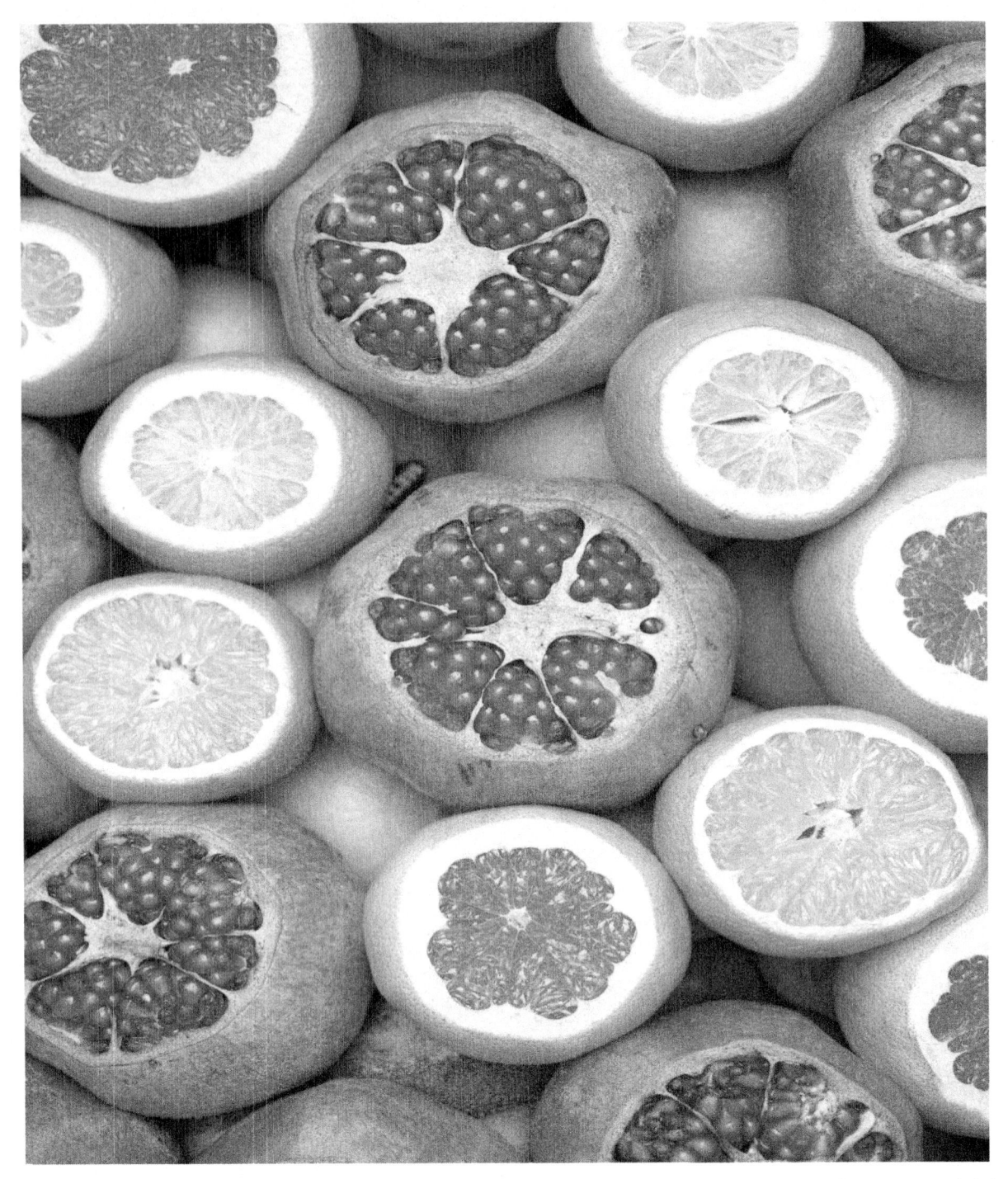

Phytochemicals, which are plant-derived compounds, have also shown tremendous potential in inhibiting cancer growth. For example, resveratrol found in grapes and red wine, has been found to have anti-cancer effects in various types of cancer, including breast, colon, and prostate cancer. Some phytochemicals, such as epigallocatechin gallate (EGCG) found in green tea, have been shown to inhibit the growth of cancer cells by targeting specific molecular pathways.

In addition to their direct anti-cancer effects, nutraceuticals may also have a role to play in enhancing the effectiveness of traditional cancer treatments. For example, some studies have shown that polyphenols and other nutraceuticals can increase the sensitivity of cancer cells to chemotherapy and radiation therapy, making these treatments more effective.

While the use of nutraceuticals as metabolic therapeutics for cancer is still in its early stages, there is growing evidence to support their potential role in the prevention and treatment of cancer. However, it is important to note that the effectiveness and safety of these compounds may vary depending on the type and stage of cancer, as well as individual factors such as diet and lifestyle.

The field of nutraceuticals as metabolic therapeutics for cancer is a promising one, offering new strategies for preventing and treating this devastating disease. However, further research is needed to fully understand their mechanisms of action and potential side effects. With continued research and clinical trials, nutraceuticals may become an important addition to the arsenal of tools for fighting cancer and improving overall health and wellbeing.

Chapter 5: The role of fasting and calorie restriction in cancer treatment: examining the effects of reducing calorie intake on cancer cell metabolism and tumor growth

Fasting and calorie restriction have long been used in various religious and spiritual practices, but recent studies have shown that they may also have benefits in cancer treatment. Cancer is a complex disease where cells grow uncontrollably, leading to the formation of tumors. These abnormal cells have a different metabolism compared to normal cells and require a high amount of energy to support their rapid growth. This is where the role of fasting and calorie restriction comes into play.

In simple terms, fasting involves voluntarily abstaining from food or drink for a certain period of time. On the other hand, calorie restriction is a controlled reduction in calorie intake, typically by 20-30% of the usual intake. Both methods cause a state of nutrient deprivation in the body, which has a direct impact on cancer cells.

Several studies have shown that fasting and calorie restriction can inhibit tumor growth and improve the efficacy of cancer treatments. One of the reasons behind this is that cancer cells have a high demand for glucose, the body's main source of energy. In a state of deprivation, the body switches to using other energy sources, such as fats and ketones, which cancer cells are not able to utilize efficiently. This leads to a decrease in the energy supply for cancer cells, ultimately hindering their growth.

Furthermore, studies have also shown that fasting and calorie restriction can increase the effectiveness of chemotherapy and radiation therapy. Cancer treatments work by targeting the fast-dividing cancer cells, but these therapies often have negative effects on healthy cells as well. Calorie restriction has been found to protect healthy cells from these treatments, while cancer cells are more vulnerable due to their high energy demand.

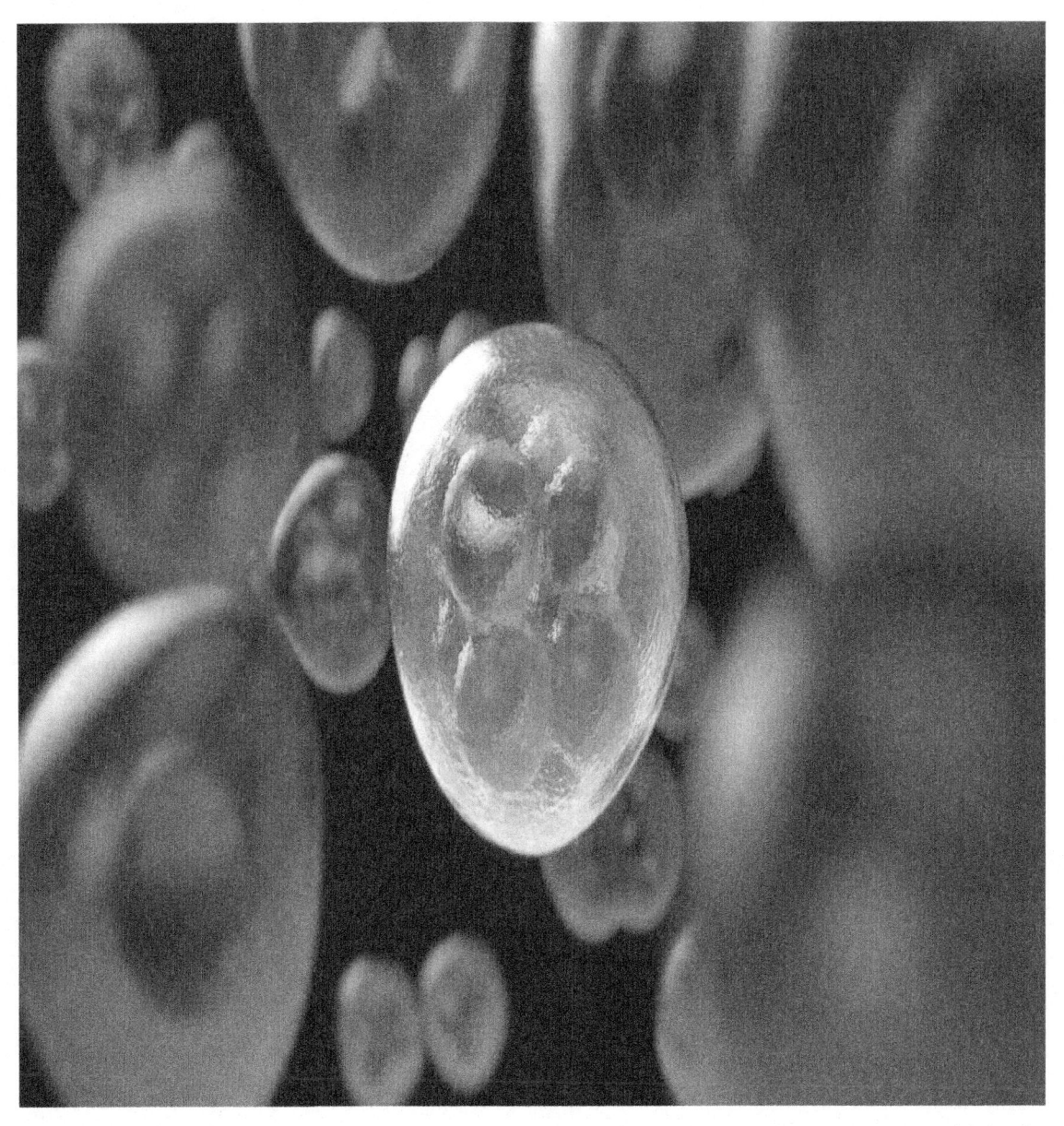

Fasting and calorie restriction also have an impact on the body's immune system, which plays a crucial role in fighting cancer. When nutrient deprivation occurs, the body initiates a process called autophagy, where old and damaged cells are cleared out and replaced with new ones. This process helps in strengthening the immune system and getting rid of any precancerous cells that may be present.

Moreover, fasting and calorie restriction have also been found to have direct effects on the genes involved in cancer development. They can influence the expression of genes related to cell growth, repair, and inflammation, all of which play a role in cancer development. By fasting or reducing calorie intake, these genes can be regulated, potentially slowing down cancer growth.

However, it is important to note that fasting and calorie restriction should always be done under the guidance of a healthcare professional. Cancer patients undergoing treatment may already have weakened immune systems, and severe calorie restriction or long-term fasting can further compromise their health. It is essential for patients to discuss these methods with their doctors before incorporating them into their treatment plan.

In conclusion, fasting and calorie restriction have shown promising results in inhibiting cancer growth and enhancing the effectiveness of cancer treatments. While more research is needed to fully understand the mechanisms behind these effects, it is clear that these methods have a role to play in cancer treatment. With proper medical supervision, fasting and calorie restriction may be utilized as adjunct treatments to help fight cancer and improve the overall health of patients.

Chapter 6: Metabolic therapies for cancer: an in-depth look at treatments such as hyperthermia, photodynamic therapy, and hyperbaric oxygen therapy and their impact on cancer metabolism

Cancer is a complex and multifaceted disease that manifests through uncontrolled cell growth and proliferation. Traditional cancer treatments such as chemotherapy, radiation, and surgery have been the primary methods of intervention for many years. However, these treatments often have significant side effects and do not target the underlying metabolic abnormalities that contribute to cancer development and progression.

Metabolic therapies for cancer offer a promising approach to treat the disease by targeting the metabolic pathways of cancer cells. These treatments aim to disrupt the unique metabolic characteristics of cancer cells, which differ significantly from healthy cells, to halt their growth and promote cell death. Some of the most promising metabolic therapies for cancer include hyperthermia, photodynamic therapy, and hyperbaric oxygen therapy.

Hyperthermia is a treatment that involves raising the body's temperature to kill cancer cells. It works by targeting cancer cells and reducing oxygen supply, which they require in higher amounts compared to normal cells. This treatment can be performed by either external or internal hyperthermia. In external hyperthermia, the tumor is exposed to an external energy source, such as microwaves, to raise its temperature. On the other hand, internal hyperthermia involves the insertion of catheters, probes, or needles into the tumor and using them to deliver heat directly.

One of the main advantages of hyperthermia is the ability to target cancer cells while sparing healthy cells. This is because cancer cells have a weaker ability to adapt to temperature changes, making them more vulnerable to the heat. Hyperthermia also works synergistically with other treatments, such as chemotherapy and radiation, making it a suitable adjuvant therapy. Additionally, hyperthermia can enhance the immune system, stimulate blood flow, and improve the delivery of oxygen and nutrients to the tumor, making it more susceptible to other treatments.

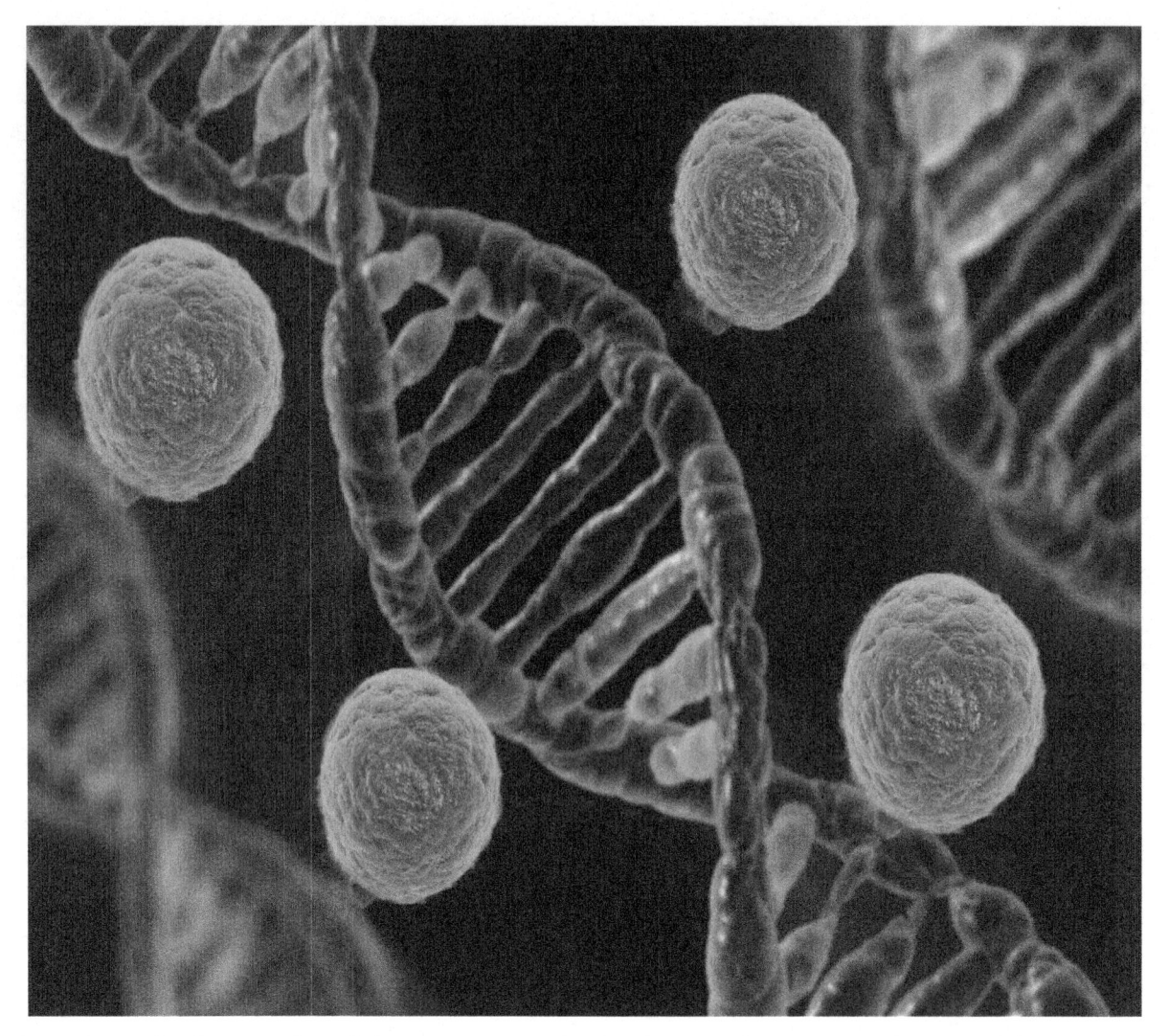

Photodynamic therapy (PDT) is another metabolic therapy that uses a photosensitizer, a light-sensitive compound, to generate reactive oxygen species (ROS) within cancer cells. These ROS cause significant damage to cancer cell membranes and lead to cell death. The photosensitizer is injected into the body and allowed to accumulate in tumor cells. Once the photosensitizer is activated by light, it releases energy in the form of ROS, which specifically target and destroy cancer cells.

PDT has several advantages over traditional cancer therapies. It is minimally invasive, allows for precise targeting, and has fewer side effects. Moreover, PDT can be repeated if necessary, and it does not cause resistance in cancer cells. It also shows promising results when used in combination with other treatments, such as chemotherapy and radiation.

Hyperbaric oxygen therapy (HBOT) involves breathing pure oxygen in a high-pressure chamber. The increased pressure in the chamber allows for a greater amount of oxygen to be dissolved in the body's tissues, including the tumor. Cancer cells often reside in a low-oxygen (hypoxic) environment, and by exposing them to high levels of oxygen, their growth can be inhibited.

HBOT can increase oxygen levels in the tumor, making it more susceptible to other treatments, such as radiation therapy. It can also reduce inflammation and promote the growth of new blood vessels, aiding in tissue repair and healing. Additionally, high levels of oxygen can enhance the immune system's functioning, helping the body fight against cancer cells.

Studies have shown the potential benefits of HBOT for cancer treatment, particularly in combination with other therapies. However, more research is needed to determine its safety and effectiveness in different types of cancer.

Metabolic therapies for cancer hold promise as a more targeted and effective approach to treating the disease. Hyperthermia, photodynamic therapy, and hyperbaric oxygen therapy all target the unique metabolic characteristics of cancer cells and can enhance the effectiveness of traditional treatments. While these therapies are still being studied, they offer hope for more personalized and less toxic cancer treatment options in the future.

Read more books by Caroline Johnson
You can fight cancer
How to Starve breast cancer
Recipes for delicious christmas meals
Grow your mind
Teenage Sexuality

Chapter 7: The microbiome and cancer: the influence of gut bacteria on metabolism and potential for targeted treatments

The microbiome, or the collection of microorganisms living in and on the human body, has gained increasing attention in recent years for its role in various diseases and overall health. One area of particular interest is its influence on cancer development and treatment. Research has shown that the gut microbiome plays a crucial role in modulating metabolism and immune responses, which can impact the development and progression of cancer.

The gut microbiome is a diverse and complex ecosystem, consisting of trillions of bacteria, viruses, fungi, and other microorganisms. These microbes are primarily found in the large intestine and have important functions in digestion, absorption of nutrients, and protection against harmful pathogens. They also produce metabolites, including short-chain fatty acids, which can affect various processes in the body. For example, some metabolites have been found to have anti-inflammatory properties, while others can promote the growth of cancer cells.

Studies have shown that certain patterns of the gut microbiome can increase the risk of developing certain types of cancer. For example, individuals with a high abundance of certain types of gut bacteria, such as Bacteroides fragilis, have been found to have an increased risk of colorectal cancer. This may be due to the production of toxins by these bacteria or their ability to alter the gut environment, leading to inflammation and damage to the intestinal lining.

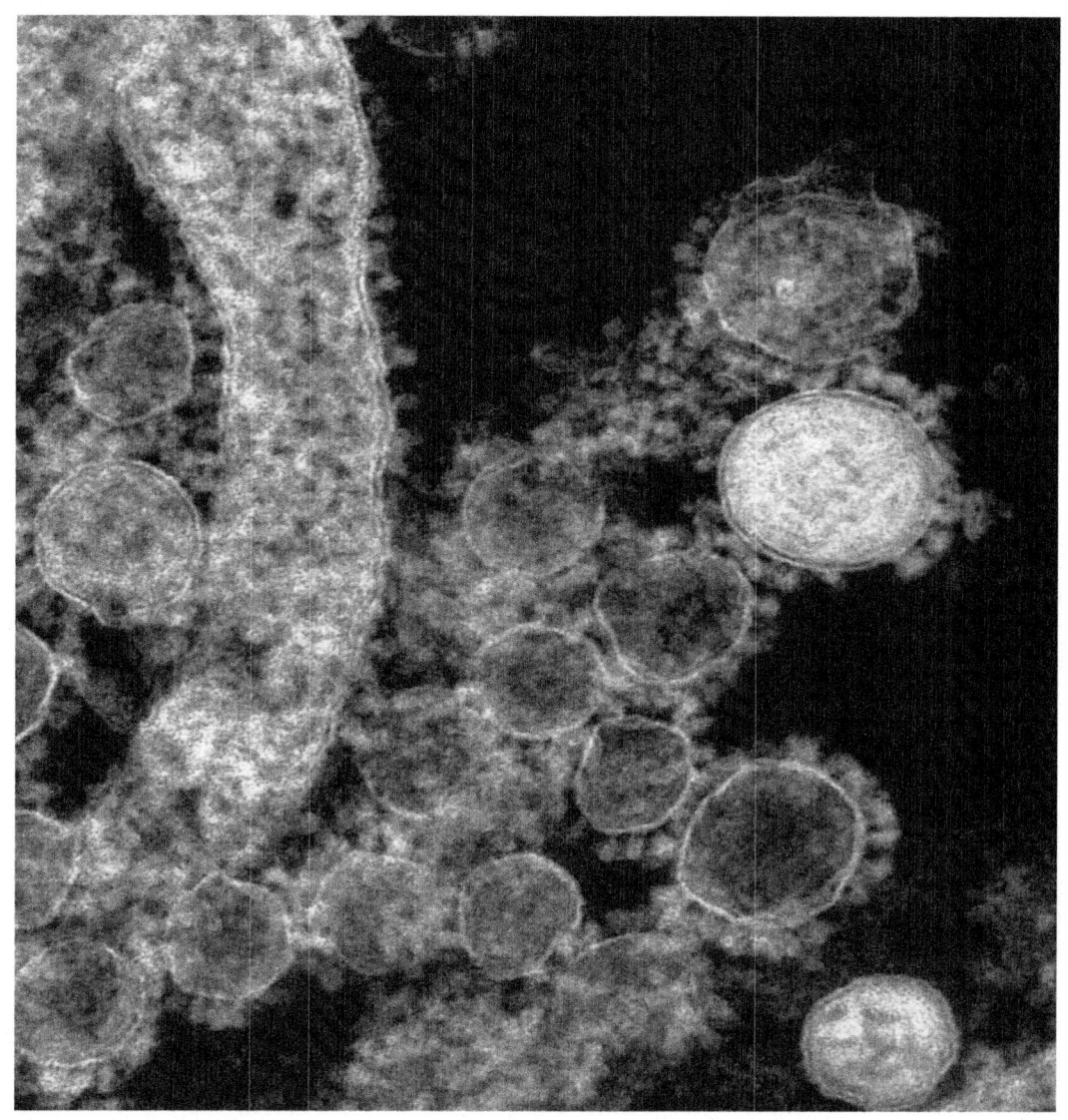

Additionally, the gut microbiome has been found to influence the efficacy and toxicity of cancer treatments. Chemotherapy, for example, can disrupt the balance of the gut microbiome, leading to changes in metabolism and immune function. This disruption can also contribute to the common side effects of chemotherapy, such as intestinal inflammation and diarrhea. On the other hand, certain types of bacteria have been found to enhance the effects of chemotherapy, suggesting a possible role for targeted thempumbiome-based therapies in cancer treatment.

Some emerging research also suggests that the microbiome can impact the responsiveness to immunotherapy, a type of cancer treatment that boosts the body's immune system to recognize and target cancer cells. A study found that patients with melanoma who responded well to immunotherapy had a more diverse gut microbiome compared to non-responders. This indicates that the gut microbiome may play a critical role in modulating the body's immune response to cancer.

The potential for using the microbiome to improve cancer treatment has led to the development of targeted therapies that aim to manipulate the gut microbiome. One approach is fecal microbiota transplantation, which involves transferring fecal material from a healthy donor to a patient in order to restore the balance of the gut microbiome. This has been tested in clinical trials for various types of cancer and has shown promising results.

Another method involves using probiotics, which are live microorganisms that can confer health benefits when consumed. Preclinical studies have shown that certain probiotic strains can inhibit the growth of cancer cells and enhance the effects of cancer treatments. However, more research is needed to fully understand how these probiotics can be used to target specific types of cancer.

The gut microbiome plays a significant role in shaping metabolism and immune responses, which can impact cancer development and treatment. Understanding the interactions between the microbiome and cancer can lead to the development of targeted therapies that can potentially improve treatment outcomes and reduce side effects. However, much more research is needed in this field to fully comprehend the potential and limitations of the microbiome in cancer prevention and treatment.

Chapter 8: Mitochondrial dysfunction in cancer cells: understanding the role of dysfunctional mitochondria in cancer development and exploring potential therapies targeting these organelles

Mitochondria are essential organelles responsible for generating energy in the form of ATP through oxidative phosphorylation. However, in cancer cells, these powerhouses undergo significant changes, leading to mitochondrial dysfunction. This altered mitochondrial function has been recognized as a hallmark of cancer, and recent studies have highlighted its crucial role in cancer development and progression.

Mitochondrial dysfunction in cancer cells is a complex process that involves various alterations in the structure, function, and metabolism of these organelles. These changes often result from metabolic reprogramming in cancer cells, which favor aerobic glycolysis over oxidative phosphorylation, a phenomenon known as the Warburg effect. The increased glycolytic activity in cancer cells leads to reduced mitochondrial respiration and ATP production, resulting in a state of energy depletion. This depletion of energy is thought to be a driving force for cancer cells to acquire mutations and adapt to harsh environments, contributing to their aggressive behavior and resistance to therapies.

One of the most well-studied alterations in mitochondrial function in cancer cells is the disruption of the electron transport chain (ETC). The ETC is a series of protein complexes located in the inner membrane of mitochondria that work together to transport electrons and generate a proton gradient across the membrane, which is essential for ATP production. In cancer cells, mutations in ETC genes and changes in the expression of ETC proteins have been reported, leading to impaired electron transport and reduced ATP production. This disruption of the ETC also results in the overproduction of reactive oxygen species (ROS), which contribute to genomic instability and promote cancer progression.

Mitochondrial DNA (mtDNA), which encodes essential genes for mitochondrial function, is also frequently mutated in cancer cells. These mutations can alter mitochondrial structure and function, impairing oxidative phosphorylation and increasing the production of ROS. Additionally, studies have shown that mtDNA mutations can lead to changes in cell metabolism, promote tumor growth, and contribute to treatment resistance.

The role of dysfunctional mitochondria in cancer has opened up new opportunities for targeted cancer therapies. Several studies have explored the use of compounds that specifically target and disrupt mitochondrial function in cancer cells. One of the most promising strategies is to target the ETC to impair ATP production and promote cell death. Inhibitors of ETC complexes, such as metformin, have shown promising results in preclinical studies, indicating their potential as an anti-cancer therapy.

Another approach is to target the increased levels of ROS in cancer cells. Drugs that act as ROS scavengers or suppressors have been tested in various cancer models and have shown to induce cell death and inhibit cancer cell growth. These therapies aim to restore the balance of ROS levels in cancer cells, leading to cell death and sensitizing tumors to other treatments.

In summary, mitochondrial dysfunction plays a critical role in cancer development and progression. The dysregulation of mitochondrial function in cancer cells leads to altered metabolism, increased ROS production, and impaired energy production, promoting cancer growth and resistance to therapy. Further understanding of the molecular mechanisms underlying mitochondrial dysfunction in cancer could lead to the development of more effective and targeted therapies for this devastating disease

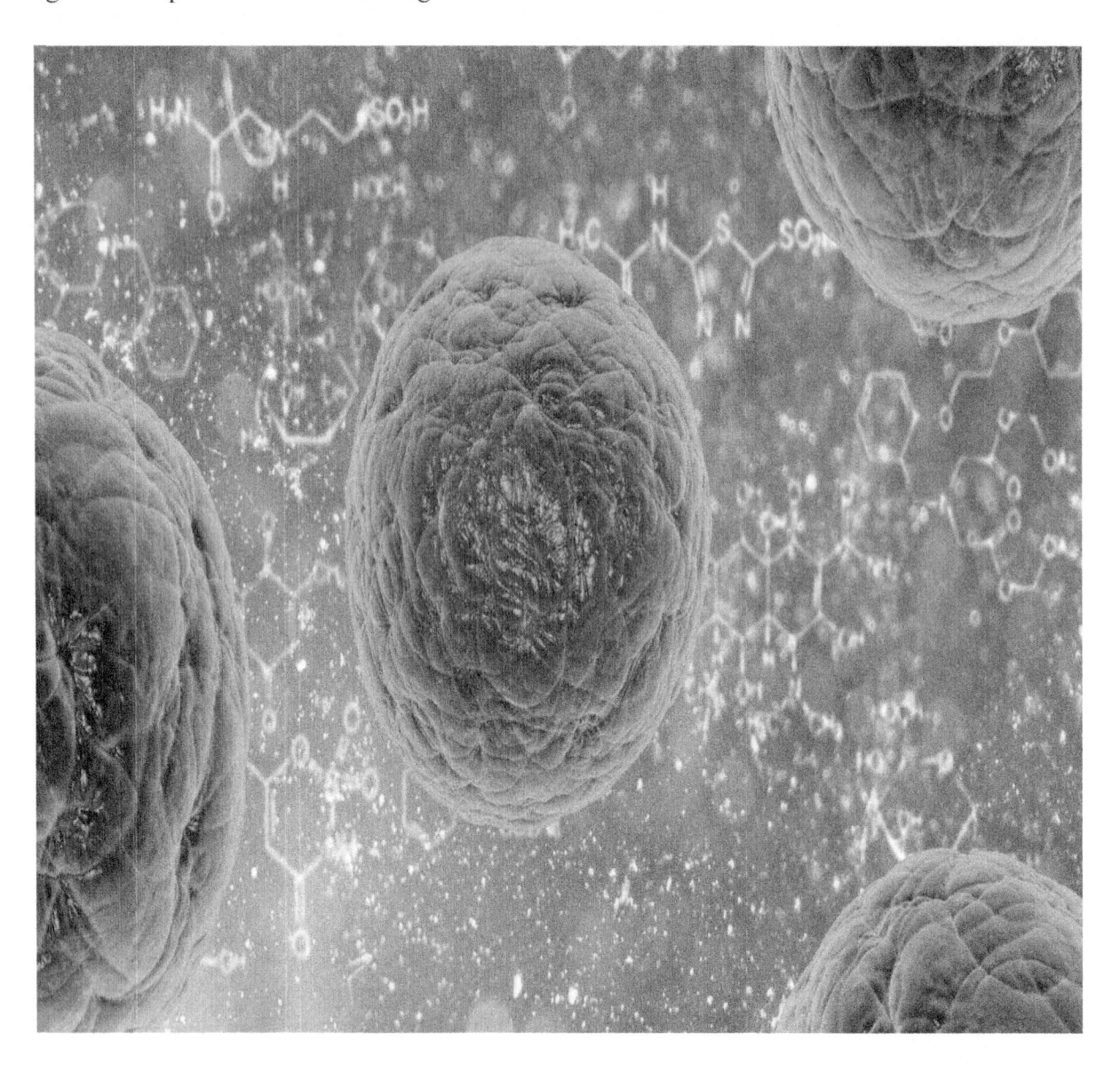

Chapter 9: Integrative approaches to cancer treatment: the combination of conventional cancer treatments with metabolic interventions for a holistic approach to healing

Integrative cancer treatments are a complementary approach to conventional cancer treatments that aim to provide a holistic approach to healing. These treatments include the combination of standard cancer treatments, such as chemotherapy, surgery, and radiation, with metabolic interventions, such as nutrition, exercise, and stress-reduction techniques.

Cancer is a complex disease, and its treatment can be equally complex. Conventional cancer treatments, such as chemotherapy and radiation, can be effective in killing cancer cells, but they can also cause significant side effects and damage healthy cells in the process. On the other hand, metabolic interventions, also known as lifestyle interventions, address the body's physiological imbalances and promote overall health and well-being, which can aid in cancer prevention and treatment.

Integrative cancer treatments bring together the best of both worlds to create a comprehensive approach to cancer management. These treatments focus on not only killing cancer cells but also on supporting the body's immune system and overall health. Metabolic interventions can help to reduce the side effects of conventional treatments, improve treatment outcomes, and improve overall quality of life.

One of the key components of integrative cancer treatment is nutrition. Nutrition plays a vital role in a cancer patient's overall health and treatment outcome. A diet that includes a variety of whole foods, such as fruits, vegetables, whole grains, and healthy fats, can help to support the body's immune system and promote healing. Additionally, some foods have been shown to have anti-cancer properties and can be incorporated into a patient's diet to support conventional treatment methods.

Exercise is another essential aspect of metabolic interventions in cancer treatment. Regular physical activity helps to improve the body's healing response and can reduce the risk of recurrence. Exercise can also alleviate cancer-related fatigue, which is a common side effect of conventional treatments.

Stress reduction techniques, such as meditation, yoga, and acupuncture, can also be effective in managing the physical and emotional symptoms of cancer treatment. These practices can help to reduce stress, anxiety, and depression, which are common in cancer patients. By managing these emotional side effects, patients can better cope with their treatment and improve their overall well-being.

Integrative cancer treatments also include alternative therapies, such as herbal supplements, acupuncture, and massage therapy. These approaches, when used in combination with conventional treatments, can help to manage side effects and improve quality of life.

By combining conventional cancer treatments with metabolic interventions, patients can benefit from a well-rounded approach to healing. Integrative treatments can improve treatment outcomes, reduce side effects, and promote overall health and well-being.

Write about Integrative approaches to cancer treatment: the combination of conventional cancer treatments with metabolic interventions for a holistic approach to healing

Integrative cancer treatments are a complementary approach to conventional cancer treatments that aim to provide a holistic approach to healing. These treatments include the combination of standard cancer treatments, such as chemotherapy, surgery, and radiation, with metabolic interventions, such as nutrition, exercise, and stress-reduction techniques.

Cancer is a complex disease, and its treatment can be equally complex. Conventional cancer treatments, such as chemotherapy and radiation, can be effective in killing cancer cells, but they can also cause significant side effects and damage healthy cells in the process. On the other hand, metabolic interventions, also known as lifestyle interventions, address the body's physiological imbalances and promote overall health and well-being, which can aid in cancer prevention and treatment.

Integrative cancer treatments bring together the best of both worlds to create a comprehensive approach to cancer management. These treatments focus on not only killing cancer cells but also on supporting the body's immune system and overall health. Metabolic interventions can help to reduce the side effects of conventional treatments, improve treatment outcomes, and improve overall quality of life.

One of the key components of integrative cancer treatment is nutrition. Nutrition plays a vital role in a cancer patient's overall health and treatment outcome. A diet that includes a variety of whole foods, such as fruits, vegetables, whole grains, and healthy fats, can help to support the body's immune system and promote healing. Additionally, some foods have been shown to have anti-cancer properties and can be incorporated into a patient's diet to support conventional treatment methods.

Exercise is another essential aspect of metabolic interventions in cancer treatment. Regular physical activity helps to improve the body's healing response and can reduce the risk of recurrence. Exercise can also alleviate cancer-related fatigue, which is a common side effect of conventional treatments.

Stress reduction techniques, such as meditation, yoga, and acupuncture, can also be effective in managing the physical and emotional symptoms of cancer treatment. These practices can help to reduce stress, anxiety, and depression, which are common in cancer patients. By managing these emotional side effects, patients can better cope with their treatment and improve their overall well-being.

Integrative cancer treatments also include alternative therapies, such as herbal supplements, acupuncture, and massage therapy. These approaches, when used in combination with conventional treatments, can help to manage side effects and improve quality of life.

By combining conventional cancer treatments with metabolic interventions, patients can benefit from a well-rounded approach to healing. Integrative treatments can improve treatment outcomes, reduce side effects, and promote overall health and well-being.

However, it is crucial to note that integrative cancer treatments should always be discussed with a healthcare provider. While these interventions can be beneficial, they should not be seen as a replacement for conventional treatment methods. It's essential to work with a medical professional to create an individualized treatment plan that includes both conventional treatments and metabolic interventions.

In conclusion, integrative cancer treatments offer a more comprehensive and holistic approach to cancer management. By combining conventional treatments with metabolic interventions, patients can receive the benefits of both approaches while supporting their body's natural healing processes.

Chapter 10: Clinical trials and future directions: reviewing current research on the metabolic approach to cancer treatment and potential directions for future studies

The metabolic approach to cancer treatment has gained significant attention in recent years as a promising alternative to traditional cancer therapies. This approach focuses on targeting the altered metabolism of cancer cells, which is characterized by increased glucose uptake and reliance on glycolysis for energy production. By inhibiting specific metabolic pathways, it is hypothesized that cancer cells can be effectively deprived of their energy source and potentially induce tumor regression.

Numerous preclinical studies have demonstrated the efficacy of the metabolic approach in various types of cancers, including breast, lung, colon, and prostate cancers. For instance, in breast cancer, inhibition of fatty acid synthesis has shown to be effective in reducing tumor growth and promoting tumor cell death. In lung cancer, targeting the glutamine metabolism has also shown promising results in reducing tumor cell proliferation and inducing cell death.

In addition to these preclinical studies, several clinical trials have also been conducted to evaluate the effectiveness of the metabolic approach in cancer treatment. A phase 1 clinical trial using the glycolysis inhibitor 2-deoxyglucose (2-DG) showed promising results in patients with advanced solid tumors, with a 50% response rate. Another phase 1 trial using the glutamine antagonist CB-839 also showed promising results in patients with solid tumors, with some patients experiencing 70% tumor shrinkage.

Despite these promising results, there are still significant challenges and limitations that need to be addressed in order for the metabolic approach to become a widely accepted cancer treatment. One major limitation is the potential for off-target effects and toxicity due to the essential role of these metabolic pathways in normal cell functioning. To overcome this, further research is needed to develop more specific and targeted inhibitors that can effectively block cancer cell metabolism without affecting normal cells.

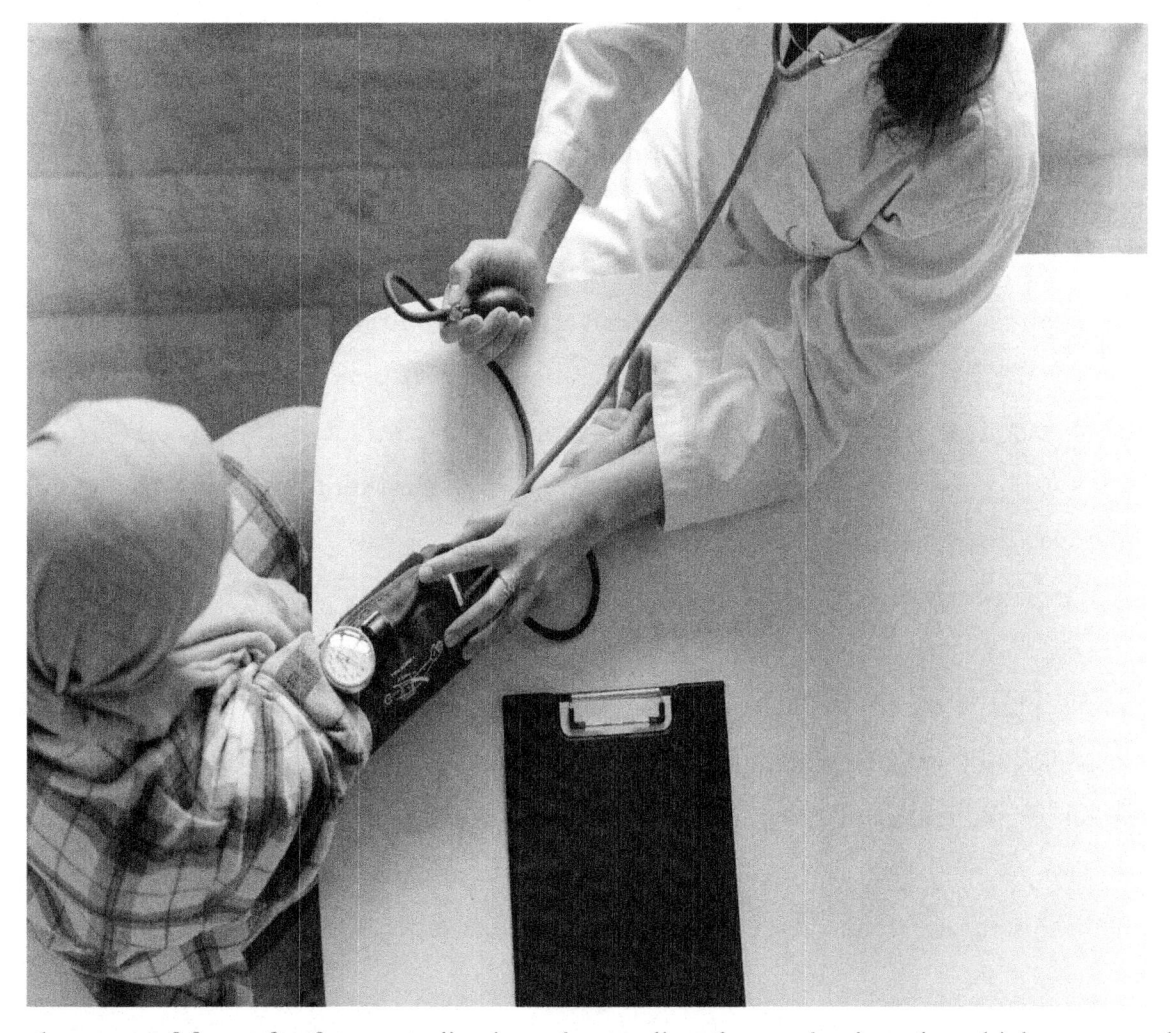

Another area of focus for future studies is understanding the mechanisms by which cancer cells develop resistance to metabolic inhibitors. This is especially important as studies have shown that cancer cells can adapt and rewire their metabolic pathways to survive under conditions of metabolic stress. By understanding these mechanisms, researchers can develop strategies to prevent or overcome resistance and improve the overall effectiveness of the metabolic approach.

Furthermore, more research is needed to better understand the role of the tumor microenvironment in cancer metabolism and treatment response. The complex interaction between cancer cells and their surrounding microenvironment can influence metabolic changes and adaptation, potentially affecting the success of metabolic therapies. Understanding the role of the tumor microenvironment in cancer metabolism can help guide the development of more effective therapeutic strategies.

In addition, there is a need for larger and more in-depth clinical trials to evaluate the effectiveness of metabolic inhibitors in Write about trials and future directions: reviewing current research on the metabolic approach to cancer treatment and potential directions for future studies.

The metabolic approach to cancer treatment has gained significant attention in recent years as a promising alternative to traditional cancer therapies. This approach focuses on targeting the altered metabolism of cancer cells, which is characterized by increased glucose uptake and reliance on glycolysis for energy production. By inhibiting specific metabolic pathways, it is hypothesized that cancer cells can be effectively deprived of their energy source and potentially induce tumor regression.

Numerous preclinical studies have demonstrated the efficacy of the metabolic approach in various types of cancers, including breast, lung, colon, and prostate cancers. For instance, in breast cancer, inhibition of fatty acid synthesis has shown to be effective in reducing tumor growth and promoting tumor cell death. In lung cancer, targeting the glutamine metabolism has also shown promising results in reducing tumor cell proliferation and inducing cell death.

In addition to these preclinical studies, several clinical trials have also been conducted to evaluate the effectiveness of the metabolic approach in cancer treatment. A phase 1 clinical trial using the glycolysis inhibitor 2-deoxyglucose (2-DG) showed promising results in patients with advanced solid tumors, with a 50% response rate. Another phase 1 trial using the glutamine antagonist CB-839 also showed promising results in patients with solid tumors, with some patients experiencing 70% tumor shrinkage.

Despite these promising results, there are still significant challenges and limitations that need to be addressed in order for the metabolic approach to become a widely accepted cancer treatment. One major limitation is the potential for off-target effects and toxicity due to the essential role of these metabolic pathways in normal cell functioning. To overcome this, further research is needed to develop more specific and targeted inhibitors that can effectively block cancer cell metabolism without affecting normal cells.

Another area of focus for future studies is understanding the mechanisms by which cancer cells develop resistance to metabolic inhibitors. This is especially important as studies have shown that cancer cells can adapt and rewire their metabolic pathways to survive under conditions of metabolic stress. By understanding these mechanisms, researchers can develop strategies to prevent or overcome resistance and improve the overall effectiveness of the metabolic approach.

Furthermore, more research is needed to better understand the role of the tumor microenvironment in cancer metabolism and treatment response. The complex interaction between cancer cells and their surrounding microenvironment can influence metabolic changes and adaptation, potentially affecting the success of metabolic therapies. Understanding the role of the tumor microenvironment in cancer metabolism can help guide the development of more effective therapeutic strategies.

In addition, there is a need for larger and more in-depth clinical trials to evaluate the effectiveness of metabolic inhibitors in different types of cancers and in combination with other therapies. This will help to establish the optimal dosage, treatment schedule, and patient selection criteria for the metabolic approach.

In conclusion, while the metabolic approach to cancer treatment has shown promising results in preclinical and early clinical studies, there are still significant challenges and limitations that need to be addressed. More research is needed to develop targeted and specific inhibitors, understand the mechanisms of resistance, and evaluate the role of the tumor microenvironment in treatment response. With continued research and advancements in technology, the metabolic approach has the potential to revolutionize cancer treatment and improve outcomes for patients.

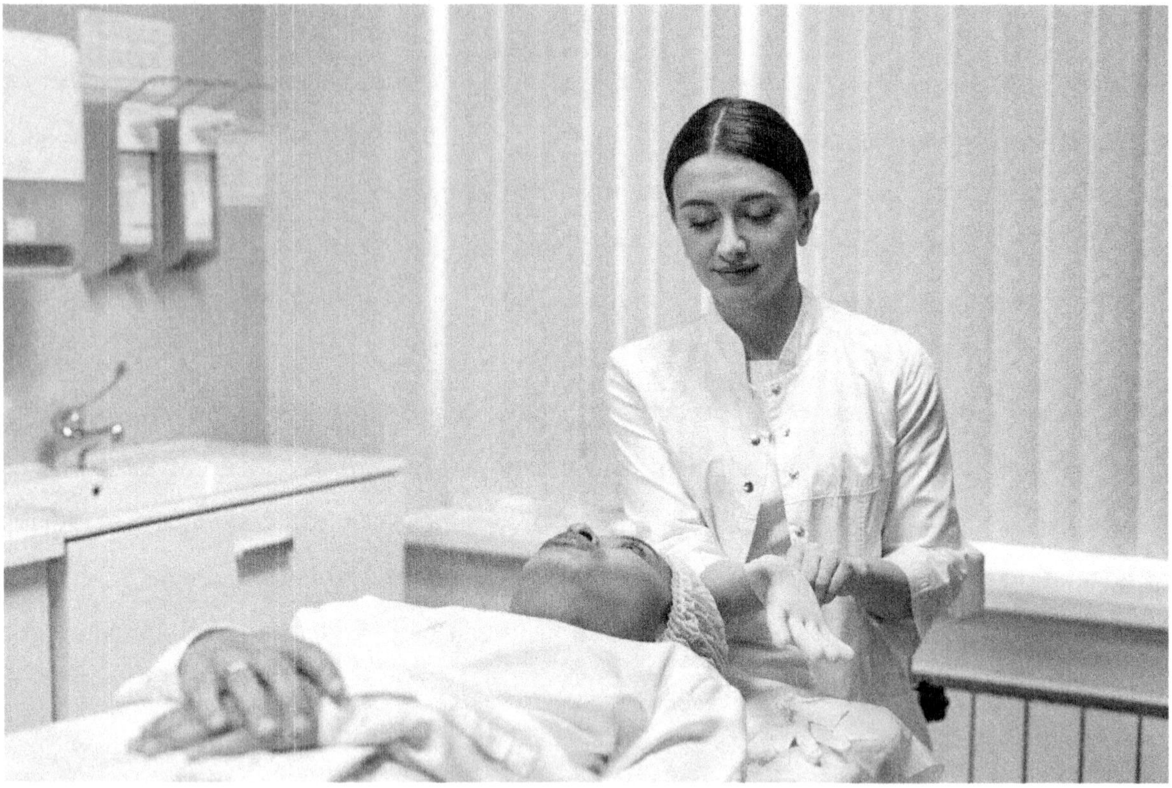

Conclusion

In conclusion, the metabolic way to heal cancer, also known as metabolic therapy, is an innovative approach that focuses on targeting the natural metabolic processes of cancer cells. By altering their energy metabolism, this therapy intends to disrupt the growth and survival of cancer cells. While traditional treatment methods such as chemotherapy and radiation therapy have shown some success in managing cancer, they often come with severe side effects. The metabolic way of healing offers a more personalized and less toxic alternative, making it a promising avenue for cancer treatment.

However, it is important to note that more research is needed to fully understand the effectiveness and safety of this approach. Nonetheless, the metabolic way to heal cancer presents a promising step towards finding a more effective and less harmful treatment for this devastating disease. With continued advancements and research, there is hope that this approach could one day revolutionize the field of cancer treatment and bring new hope to patients and their loved ones.

while the metabolic approach to cancer treatment has shown promising results in preclinical and early clinical studies, there are still significant challenges and limitations that need to be addressed. More research is needed to develop targeted and specific inhibitors, understand the mechanisms of resistance, and evaluate the role of the tumor microenvironment in treatment response. With continued research and advancements in technology, the metabolic approach has the potential to revolutionize cancer treatment and improve outcomes for patients.

Printed in Great Britain
by Amazon